MY WELLNESS
JOURNAL

_____

Name

_____

Date

3 things I am most grateful for:

1. _____

_____

_____

2. _____

_____

_____

3. _____

_____

_____

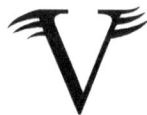

First edition 2024

Paperback ISBN: 978-1-956856-64-4

Library of Congress Control Number: 2024925926

Published by thewordverve (www.thewordverve.com)
Canton, GA, USA

Cover and print interior design by Robin Krauss
www.bookformatters.com

GUIDE TO SECTIONS IN THIS JOURNAL

The Benefits of a Journal   1

How This Journal will Help You Reach Your Welness Goals   1

How to Use This Journal   2

Collaboration with Doctors and Wellness Professionals   3

Current Health Overview   4

Wheel of Life   6

Prescription Medication   7

Over-the-Counter Medicine   10

Physician and Practitioner Directory   13

Appointments and Visits   18

Supplements Log   27

Integrative Therapies   33

Excercise Journal   37

Sleep Journal   38

Recommendations and Resources   40

Reflections and Insights   44

Emergency Information   47

Emotional and Mental Health Tracking   48

Social and Support Networks   53

Gratitude and Mindfulness   59

Environmental and Lifestyle Factors   63

Spiritual Health and Practices   67

Successes and Celebrations   70

Monthly Action Plan   72

MY WELLNESS
JOURNAL

Welcome to *My Wellness Journal*—a personalized guide designed to support you on your path to optimal health and well-being. This journal is more than just a place to record your daily activities; it is a comprehensive companion that empowers you to take control of your health, track your progress, and make informed decisions that align with your wellness goals.

The Benefits of a Journal

In today's fast-paced world, maintaining good health requires more than just occasional checkups or sporadic healthy choices. True wellness is a continuous journey that involves mindful attention to every aspect of your life—physical, mental, emotional, and spiritual. This journal is created to help you navigate this journey with intention and clarity. Your life matters, and no amount of "I'm too busy" will buy you one more minute of health. It is that important!

Whether you're managing a chronic condition, looking to improve your vitality and longevity, exploring integrative and holistic practices, or simply seeking to improve your overall well-being, this journal provides a structured space to record, reflect, and refine your approach to health.

How This Journal Will Help You Reach Your Wellness Goals

- **Comprehensive Health Tracking:** Keep a detailed record of your current health status, medications, supplements, therapies, and treatments, allowing you to see patterns, identify what's working, and make necessary adjustments.

- **Notes for Doctors Appointments:** In this crazy, busy world, it is difficult to remember all the details of your health journey. Relax and know that you have the information needed to share with your medical professionals. They can help you when they know the complete picture.

- **Goal Setting and Reflection:** Set clear wellness goals each month, track your progress, and reflect on your experiences. This practice helps you stay motivated and focused on your journey.

- **List of Recommendations and Resources:** One place to record all the good books, personal recommendations, social media videos, and ideas to research. Never lose track of ways to improve your well-being. They will be at your fingertips when you can sit down and investigate them.

- **Holistic Well-Being:** This journal encourages you to explore and document a wide range of health modalities—from traditional Western medicine to integrative and alternative practices—ensuring that you approach your health from a holistic perspective.

- **Mindfulness and Awareness:** Use this journal as a tool for mindfulness, helping you become more aware of how different factors—such as diet, exercise, sleep, and stress—impact your health. This awareness is the first step toward meaningful change.

- **Empowerment and Education:** As you document your health journey, you'll gain valuable insights into what contributes to your well-being. This journal also includes sections for recommendations, workshops, and learning, empowering you to continuously educate yourself and grow in your wellness journey.

How to Use This Journal

- **Daily Entries:** Regularly record your health-related activities, including medications, supplements, exercise, sleep, and mood. This daily tracking will help you stay consistent and notice trends over time.

- **Monthly Action Plans:** At the beginning of each month, set specific wellness goals, and outline your plan for achieving them. Use the end-of-month reflection to assess your progress and make adjustments for the future.

- **Reflection and Insight:** Periodically review your entries to gain insights into your health. Reflect on what's working, what's not, and how you can continue to optimize your well-being.

- **Family Meetings:** The healthiest people have the love, support, and collaboration of their family members. Sharing your journal with goals and outcomes will build personal relationships with those closest to you. We often presume others understand what we are going through, but many health issues (especially mental health) are not visible. Bring your family together by sharing each other's wellness journeys.

- **Personalization:** This journal is yours to customize. Add or modify sections to suit your unique needs and preferences. The more you make it your own, the more valuable it will become in your wellness journey.

Collaboration with Doctors and Wellness Professionals

Your health journey is a collaborative effort, and this journal will help you effectively communicate with your healthcare providers, whether they are doctors, specialists, or wellness practitioners. By keeping detailed records of your health, treatments, and experiences, you can provide your care team with accurate, up-to-date information, which is crucial for making informed decisions about your health.

How to Collaborate Using This Journal

- **Share Your Entries:** Bring this journal with you to appointments. Sharing your daily and monthly entries with your healthcare providers can give them a clearer picture of your progress, challenges, and overall well-being. This can lead to more personalized and effective care.

- **Discuss Your Goals:** Use the Monthly Action Plans to discuss your wellness goals with your doctors and wellness professionals. Their insights can help refine your goals and ensure they are safe and achievable.

- **Track Recommendations:** Document any advice or recommendations from your healthcare team in the designated sections. This ensures that you can follow through on their suggestions and track their effectiveness over time.

- **Integrative Care:** If you're working with both conventional doctors and alternative medicine practitioners, use this journal to bridge the gap between different treatment modalities. Keeping all your health information in one place helps ensure that everyone on your care team is informed and aligned with your overall health plan.

- **Follow-up and Feedback:** After implementing new treatments, medications, or lifestyle changes recommended by your care team, use this journal to track the outcomes. At your next appointment, you can discuss these notes, allowing for more informed follow-up care.

Current Health Overview

Personal Health & Wellness Snapshot

Date of Entry	
Current Weight	
Height and BMI	
Blood Pressure	
Heart	
Blood Sugar Levels	
Hemoglobin A1c	
Other blood marker numbers to track/ monitor (hormones, vitamins, etc):	

Health Goals

Short-term and long-term health goals (weight loss, improved sleep, reduced stress)

1. _____

2. _____

3. _____

Top 3 Issues to Improve

What are the top 3 problems I deal with daily? (chronic fatigue, social media addiction, etc. . . .)

1. _____

2. _____

3. _____

Top 3 Long-term Goals

What are the top 3 goals that I have for the long term? (run a marathon, climb the Acropolis in Greece, etc. . . .)

1. _____

2. _____

3. _____

Overall Well-Being

Self-assessment scale (1-10)	Least									Best
	1	2	3	4	5	6	7	8	9	10
Health (Physical)	○	○	○	○	○	○	○	○	○	○
Spiritual (Mental)	○	○	○	○	○	○	○	○	○	○
Career	○	○	○	○	○	○	○	○	○	○
Personal Development	○	○	○	○	○	○	○	○	○	○
Social Life	○	○	○	○	○	○	○	○	○	○
Finance	○	○	○	○	○	○	○	○	○	○
Friends	○	○	○	○	○	○	○	○	○	○
Family	○	○	○	○	○	○	○	○	○	○

Wheel of Life

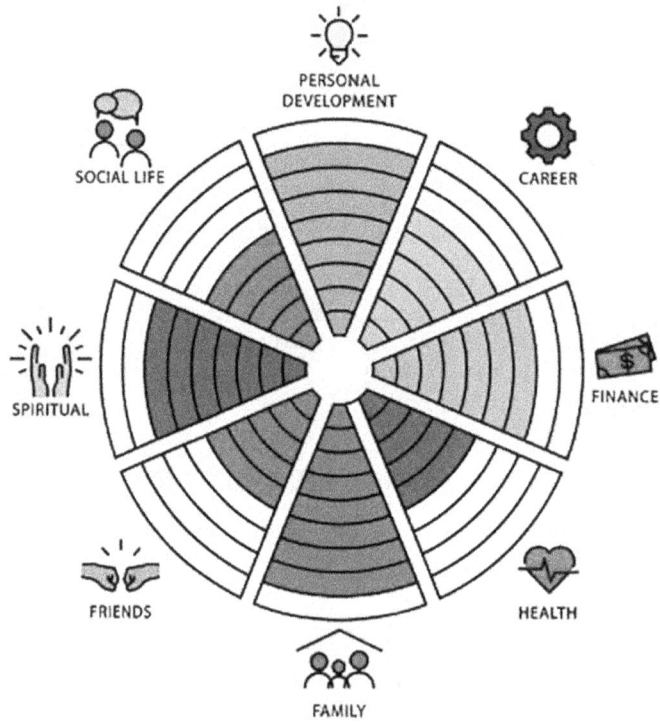

With colored markers, complete the diagram below as in the sample above according to your "Overall Well-Being" answers on the previous page.

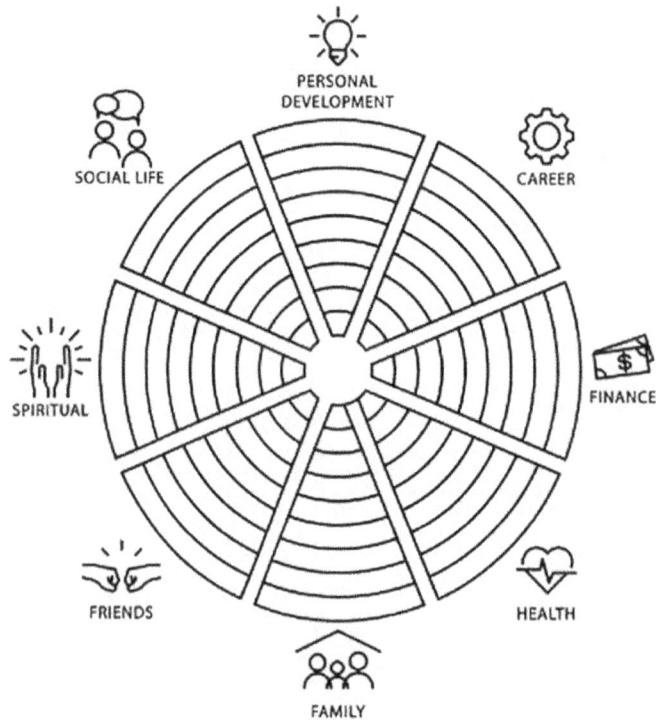

Prescription Medication

Prescription Medication	
Name of Medication	
Dosage and Frequency	
Prescribing Physician	
Start Date | End Date	
Notes on Benefits, Side Effects or Reactions	

Prescription Medication	
Name of Medication	
Dosage and Frequency	
Prescribing Physician	
Start Date | End Date	
Notes on Benefits, Side Effects or Reactions	

Prescription Medication		
Name of Medication		
Dosage and Frequency		
Prescribing Physician		
Start Date	End Date		
Notes on Benefits, Side Effects or Reactions		

Prescription Medication		
Name of Medication		
Dosage and Frequency		
Prescribing Physician		
Start Date	End Date		
Notes on Benefits, Side Effects or Reactions		

Prescription Medication		
Name of Medication		
Dosage and Frequency		
Prescribing Physician		
Start Date | End Date		
Notes on Benefits, Side Effects or Reactions		

Prescription Medication		
Name of Medication		
Dosage and Frequency		
Prescribing Physician		
Start Date | End Date		
Notes on Benefits, Side Effects or Reactions		

Over-the-Counter Medicine

Over-the-Counter Medication	
Name of Medication	
Dosage and Frequency	
Purpose for Use	
Start Date | End Date	
Notes on Effectiveness or Reactions *(visit www.drugs.com for an interaction checker)*	

Over-the-Counter Medication	
Name of Medication	
Dosage and Frequency	
Purpose for Use	
Start Date | End Date	
Notes on Effectiveness or Reactions *(visit www.drugs.com for an interaction checker)*	

Over-the-Counter Medication	
Name of Medication	
Dosage and Frequency	
Purpose for Use	
Start Date | End Date	
Notes on Effectiveness or Reactions (visit www.drugs.com for an interaction checker)	

Over-the-Counter Medication	
Name of Medication	
Dosage and Frequency	
Purpose for Use	
Start Date | End Date	
Notes on Effectiveness or Reactions (visit www.drugs.com for an interaction checker)	

Over-the-Counter Medication	
Name of Medication	
Dosage and Frequency	
Purpose for Use	
Start Date | End Date	
Notes on Effectiveness or Reactions *(visit www.drugs.com for an interaction checker)*	

Over-the-Counter Medication	
Name of Medication	
Dosage and Frequency	
Purpose for Use	
Start Date | End Date	
Notes on Effectiveness or Reactions *(visit www.drugs.com for an interaction checker)*	

Physician and Practitioner Directory

Primary Care Physician	
Name	
Contact Information	
Purpose for Use	
Notes	

Specialist	
Name	
Specialty	
Contact Information	
Notes on Visits or Treatments	

Specialist	
Name	
Specialty	
Contact Information	
Notes on Visits or Treatments	

Specialist	
Name	
Specialty	
Contact Information	
Notes on Visits or Treatments	

Integrative Medicine Practitioner	
Name	
Modality (acupuncture, chiropractic, etc....)	
Contact Information	
Notes on Visits or Treatments	

Integrative Medicine Practitioner	
Name	
Modality (acupuncture, chiropractic, etc....)	
Contact Information	
Notes on Visits or Treatments	

Wellness Practitioner	
Name	
Modality (hypnotist, Reiki practitioner, masseuse, etc. . . .)	
Contact Information	
Notes on Visits or Treatments	

Wellness Practitioner	
Name	
Modality (hypnotist, Reiki practitioner, masseuse, etc. . . .)	
Contact Information	
Notes on Visits or Treatments	

Wellness Practitioner	
Name	
Modality (hypnotist, Reiki practitioner, masseuse, etc. . . .)	
Contact Information	
Notes on Visits or Treatments	

Wellness Practitioner	
Name	
Modality (hypnotist, Reiki practitioner, masseuse, etc. . . .)	
Contact Information	
Notes on Visits or Treatments	

Appointments and Visits

Doctor's Visit	
Date of Visit	
Physician or Practitioner	
Reason for Visit	
Summary of Discussion and Recommendations	
Follow-Up Needed	◯ Yes ◯ No *(place tasks on your monthly action plan)*

▼

Lab Tests and Results	
Date of Test	
Type of Test	
Results Summary	
Notes or Actions Taken	
Follow-Up Needed	◯ Yes ◯ No *(place tasks on your monthly action plan)*

Doctor's Visit	
Date of Visit	
Physician or Practitioner	
Reason for Visit	
Summary of Discussion and Recommendations	
Follow-Up Needed	◯ Yes ◯ No *(place tasks on your monthly action plan)*

Lab Tests and Results	
Date of Test	
Type of Test	
Results Summary	
Notes or Actions Taken	
Follow-Up Needed	◯ Yes ◯ No *(place tasks on your monthly action plan)*

Doctor's Visit	
Date of Visit	
Physician or Practitioner	
Reason for Visit	
Summary of Discussion and Recommendations	
Follow-Up Needed	◯ Yes ◯ No *(place tasks on your monthly action plan)*

Lab Tests and Results	
Date of Test	
Type of Test	
Results Summary	
Notes or Actions Taken	
Follow-Up Needed	◯ Yes ◯ No *(place tasks on your monthly action plan)*

Doctor's Visit	
Date of Visit	
Physician or Practitioner	
Reason for Visit	
Summary of Discussion and Recommendations	
Follow-Up Needed	◯ Yes ◯ No *(place tasks on your monthly action plan)*

Lab Tests and Results	
Date of Test	
Type of Test	
Results Summary	
Notes or Actions Taken	
Follow-Up Needed	◯ Yes ◯ No *(place tasks on your monthly action plan)*

Doctor's Visit	
Date of Visit	
Physician or Practitioner	
Reason for Visit	
Summary of Discussion and Recommendations	
Follow-Up Needed	◯ Yes ◯ No *(place tasks on your monthly action plan)*

Lab Tests and Results	
Date of Test	
Type of Test	
Results Summary	
Notes or Actions Taken	
Follow-Up Needed	◯ Yes ◯ No *(place tasks on your monthly action plan)*

Doctor's Visit	
Date of Visit	
Physician or Practitioner	
Reason for Visit	
Summary of Discussion and Recommendations	
Follow-Up Needed	○ Yes ○ No *(place tasks on your monthly action plan)*

Lab Tests and Results	
Date of Test	
Type of Test	
Results Summary	
Notes or Actions Taken	
Follow-Up Needed	○ Yes ○ No *(place tasks on your monthly action plan)*

Doctor's Visit	
Date of Visit	
Physician or Practitioner	
Reason for Visit	
Summary of Discussion and Recommendations	
Follow-Up Needed	◯ Yes ◯ No *(place tasks on your monthly action plan)*

Lab Tests and Results	
Date of Test	
Type of Test	
Results Summary	
Notes or Actions Taken	
Follow-Up Needed	◯ Yes ◯ No *(place tasks on your monthly action plan)*

Doctor's Visit	
Date of Visit	
Physician or Practitioner	
Reason for Visit	
Summary of Discussion and Recommendations	
Follow-Up Needed	◯ Yes ◯ No *(place tasks on your monthly action plan)*

Lab Tests and Results	
Date of Test	
Type of Test	
Results Summary	
Notes or Actions Taken	
Follow-Up Needed	◯ Yes ◯ No *(place tasks on your monthly action plan)*

Immunizations and Vaccinations	
Date	
Type of Vaccine	
Notes on Reactions	

>> ATTACH PRINTOUT FROM DOCTOR HERE <<

Supplements Log

Supplement	
Name of Supplement	
Brand and Dosage	
How to take supplements (with food, without, at night, etc. . . .)	
Purpose (immunity, digestion, deficit, etc. . . .)	
Where to buy it (doctor, Amazon, other website, local store, etc.. . .)	
Start Date | End Date	
Notes on Effects or Reactions	

Supplement	
Name of Supplement	
Brand and Dosage	
How to take supplements (with food, without, at night, etc. . . .)	
Purpose (immunity, digestion, deficit, etc. . . .)	
Where to buy it (doctor, Amazon, other website, local store, etc.. . .)	
Start Date | End Date	
Notes on Effects or Reactions	

Supplement	
Name of Supplement	
Brand and Dosage	
How to take supplements (with food, without, at night, etc. . . .)	
Purpose (immunity, digestion, deficit, etc. . . .)	
Where to buy it (doctor, Amazon, other website, local store, etc. . . .)	
Start Date | End Date	
Notes on Effects or Reactions	

Supplement	
Name of Supplement	
Brand and Dosage	
How to take supplements (with food, without, at night, etc. . . .)	
Purpose (immunity, digestion, deficit, etc. . . .)	
Where to buy it (doctor, Amazon, other website, local store, etc.. . . .)	
Start Date | End Date	
Notes on Effects or Reactions	

Supplement	
Name of Supplement	
Brand and Dosage	
How to take supplements (with food, without, at night, etc. . . .)	
Purpose (immunity, digestion, deficit, etc. . . .)	
Where to buy it (doctor, Amazon, other website, local store, etc. . . .)	
Start Date | End Date	
Notes on Effects or Reactions	

Supplement	
Name of Supplement	
Brand and Dosage	
How to take supplements (with food, without, at night, etc. . . .)	
Purpose (immunity, digestion, deficit, etc. . . .)	
Where to buy it (doctor, Amazon, other website, local store, etc.. . . .)	
Start Date | End Date	
Notes on Effects or Reactions	

Integrative Therapies

Refer to The Wellness Journey: Resources for Health and Healing

Integrative Practices and Modalities

Practice	
Modality (e.g., yoga, meditation, acupuncture)	
Practitioner	
Frequency and duration	
Notes on experience and benefits	

Practice	
Modality (e.g., yoga, meditation, acupuncture)	
Practitioner	
Frequency and duration	
Notes on experience and benefits	

Practice	
Modality (e.g., yoga, meditation, acupuncture)	
Practitioner	
Frequency and duration	
Notes on experience and benefits	

Practice	
Modality (e.g., yoga, meditation, acupuncture)	
Practitioner	
Frequency and duration	
Notes on experience and benefits	

Practice	
Modality (e.g., yoga, meditation, acupuncture)	
Practitioner	
Frequency and duration	
Notes on experience and benefits	

Practice	
Modality (e.g., yoga, meditation, acupuncture)	
Practitioner	
Frequency and duration	
Notes on experience and benefits	

Practice	
Modality (e.g., yoga, meditation, acupuncture)	
Practitioner	
Frequency and duration	
Notes on experience and benefits	

Practice	
Modality (e.g., yoga, meditation, acupuncture)	
Practitioner	
Frequency and duration	
Notes on experience and benefits	

Exercise Journal

Daily/Weekly Exercise Log

Practice	
Date	
Type of exercise	
Duration	Intensity level (e.g., run 5 miles, lift 20 lbs.)
Notes on performance and feelings	

Goals and Progress

Practice	
Fitness goals (e.g., run 5 miles, lift 20 lbs.)	
Milestones achieved	
Notes on challenges or adjustments needed	
Accountability partner	

Sleep Journal

Daily Sleep Log

Date	
Time to bed and time of wakeup	
Total hours of sleep	
Sleep quality rating (1-10)	Worst Best 1 2 3 4 5 6 7 8 9 10 ◯ ◯ ◯ ◯ ◯ ◯ ◯ ◯ ◯ ◯
Notes on dreams, night wakings, or restlessness	

Sleep Improvement Goals

Goals (improve sleep quality, reduce insomnia)	
Strategies tried (no screens before bed, meditation)	
Progress and adjustments	

Sleep Study

Date	
Doctor	
Results	

Recommendations and Resources

Recommendations from Others

Book, article, or study	
Item recommended by physicians, practitioners, or friends	
Notes on why it was recommended	
Actions taken (e.g., read, implemented advice)	

Book, article, or study	
Item recommended by physicians, practitioners, or friends	
Notes on why it was recommended	
Actions taken (e.g., read, implemented advice)	

Books and Media to Explore

Title	
Author	
Summary of content	
Personal takeaways	

Title	
Author	
Summary of content	
Personal takeaways	

Course and Workshops

Name and description	
Date and location	
Notes on what was learned and applied	

Name and description	
Date and location	
Notes on what was learned and applied	

Reflections and Insights

Monthly or Quarterly Reflection
What health improvements have you noticed?
Challenges encountered and how you overcame them
New practices or habits adopted

Mindfulness and Gratitude

Daily or weekly gratitude

Mindfulness practices integrated and their effects

Looking Forward

Health goals for the next period

Changes to routine or new practices to try

Emergency Information

Emergency Contacts

Primary contact	
Name	Phone
Secondary contact	
Name	Phone

Allergies and Conditions

Known allergies	
Chronic conditions and important notes	

Medications and Dosages

Medication	Dose	Instructions
Medication	Dose	Instructions
Medication	Dose	Instructions
Medication	Dose	Instructions
Medication	Dose	Instructions
Medication	Dose	Instructions

Emotional and Mental Health Tracking

Mood Tracker

Mood Log												
Day or week	Poor	1	2	3	4	5	6	7	8	9	10	Great
		◯	◯	◯	◯	◯	◯	◯	◯	◯	◯	
Patterns and triggers												

Mood Log												
Day or week	Poor	1	2	3	4	5	6	7	8	9	10	Great
		◯	◯	◯	◯	◯	◯	◯	◯	◯	◯	
Patterns and triggers												

Mood Log												
Day or week	Poor	1	2	3	4	5	6	7	8	9	10	Great
		◯	◯	◯	◯	◯	◯	◯	◯	◯	◯	
Patterns and triggers												

Mood Log												
Day or week	Poor	1	2	3	4	5	6	7	8	9	10	Great
		◯	◯	◯	◯	◯	◯	◯	◯	◯	◯	
Patterns and triggers												

Mood Log												
Day or week	Poor	1	2	3	4	5	6	7	8	9	10	Great
		◯	◯	◯	◯	◯	◯	◯	◯	◯	◯	
Patterns and triggers												

Stress Management

Stress level tracking												
Day or week	Poor	1	2	3	4	5	6	7	8	9	10	Great
		○	○	○	○	○	○	○	○	○	○	
Coping strategies												

Stress level tracking												
Day or week	Poor	1	2	3	4	5	6	7	8	9	10	Great
		○	○	○	○	○	○	○	○	○	○	
Coping strategies												

Stress level tracking												
Day or week	Poor	1	2	3	4	5	6	7	8	9	10	Great
		○	○	○	○	○	○	○	○	○	○	
Coping strategies												

Stress level tracking												
Day or week	Poor	1	2	3	4	5	6	7	8	9	10	Great
		○	○	○	○	○	○	○	○	○	○	
Coping strategies												

Stress level tracking												
Day or week	Poor	1	2	3	4	5	6	7	8	9	10	Great
		○	○	○	○	○	○	○	○	○	○	
Coping strategies												

Mindfulness and Meditation:

Mindfulness practice	Impact on well-being
Mindfulness activities, such as meditation, gratitude, or deep breathing exercises.	How has this practice affected your overall mental and emotional health?

Social and Support Networks

Support Network

Key individuals who provide emotional, mental, or practical support (e.g., family, friends, support groups)

Contacts	
Name	Phone
Name	Phone
Name	Phone
Name	Phone
Name	Phone

Support Group Attendance

Log your tracking attendance at support groups, therapy sessions, or community meetings, along with reflections on their impact.

Date	Group
Reflections	

Date	Group
Reflections	

Date	Group
Reflections	

Date	Group
Reflections	

Date	Group
Reflections	

Date	Group
Reflections	

Date	Group
Reflections	

Community and Connection

Note significant social interactions, community involvement, or activities that fostered a sense of belonging.

Date	Activity
Reflections	

Date	Activity
Reflections	

Date	Activity
Reflections	

Date	Activity
Reflections	

Gratitude and Mindfulness

Gratitude Journal

Jot down things you're grateful for each day or week. This can be a powerful tool for enhancing mental and emotional health.

What I am grateful for

Reflect on positive experiences, accomplishments, or moments of joy that occurred during the month.

Positivity reflections

Affirmations:

Write daily affirmations or positive statements that align with your wellness goals.

Daily affirmation

Impact of affirmation

Daily affirmation

Impact of affirmation

Daily affirmation

Impact of affirmation

Daily affirmation

Impact of affirmation

Environmental and Lifestyle Factors

Living Environment

A section for users to assess their living space, focusing on factors like air quality, lighting, and organization, which can impact health.

Home environment assessment												
Air quality	Poor	1 ○	2 ○	3 ○	4 ○	5 ○	6 ○	7 ○	8 ○	9 ○	10 ○	Great
Lighting	Poor	1 ○	2 ○	3 ○	4 ○	5 ○	6 ○	7 ○	8 ○	9 ○	10 ○	Great
Organization	Poor	1 ○	2 ○	3 ○	4 ○	5 ○	6 ○	7 ○	8 ○	9 ○	10 ○	Great

Note any changes you've made to their environment to support better health (e.g., reducing clutter, adding plants, improving lighting).

Changes and improvements

Work-Life Balance

Assess how balanced your work and personal life is, along with strategies for improvement.

Poor   1   2   3   4   5   6   7   8   9   10   Great
       ◯   ◯   ◯   ◯   ◯   ◯   ◯   ◯   ◯   ◯

Strategies to improve

Time Management

Track how you spend your time each day. Identify areas where you can make adjustments to support your wellness.

Time spent on . . .	Strategies to improve

Spiritual Health and Practices

Spiritual Practices

Track your spiritual activities, such as prayer, meditation, attending religious services, or personal reflection. Reflect on how your spiritual practices influence your mental, emotional, and physical health.

Daily/Weekly spritual practice	Impact on well-being

Personal Growth

Record any spiritual lessons or insights gained during the month.

Lessons and insights

How has your wellness journey aligned with your sense of purpose or life's meaning?

Connection to Purpose

Successes and Celebrations

Monthly Achievements

Celebrate small and big wins throughout the month, whether related to health goals, personal growth, or overcoming challenges.

Milestones reached

Rewards and Recognition

Acknowledge your hard work and progress, and consider rewarding yourself with something meaningful (e.g., a treat, a day off, a new book).

Self-recognition

Monthly Action Plan

Purpose

Congratulations on participating in your wellness! This section is designed to help you plan, monitor, and adjust your wellness journey on a monthly basis. It allows for quick reference to the most important aspects of health, ensuring you stay on track with your goals and interventions. *You deserve health and vitality!*

Month _____   **Year** _____

Monthly Wellness Goals

What is your main health objective for this month?
("Improve sleep quality," "Reduce stress," "Increase physical activity")

Primary Wellness Goal

List additional goals that support your primary objective.
("Incorporate 10 minutes of meditation daily," "Walk 10,000 steps each day")

Secondary Wellness Goals	Key Motivations

Medications

Review and list all medications being taken this month. Note any changes in dosage, frequency, or new medications added. Are there specific side effects or reactions to watch for? How are you feeling on these medications?

Current Medications	Monitoring

Supplements

List all supplements being used this month, including dosage and purpose. How are these supplements affecting your health? Any noticeable benefits or side effects?

Supplements being taken	Effectiveness

Any new supplements introduced this month? Why were they added? How are these supplements affecting your health? Any noticeable benefits or side effects?

New supplements	Effectiveness

Therapies and Treatments

List any ongoing therapies (e.g., physical therapy, acupuncture, chiropractic) and their frequency.

Ongoing Therapies	Frequency

Note any new therapies or treatments you're starting this month.

New treatments

What progress have you noticed? Any areas of concern or need for adjustment?

Tracking progress

Integrative and Holistic Practices

List any integrative practices like meditation, yoga, or dietary changes you're focusing on this month.

Current practices

New Practices

List the new practices you're trying. How consistently are you practicing these methods? What are the outcomes so far? What habits can I improve on?

New practices & Constistency	Outcomes

Exercise and Physical Activity

List your planned exercise routine for the month, including types of exercise and frequency.

Exercise	Frequency

Track your progress toward fitness goals and note any adjustments needed to your routine.

Progress	Adjustments

What challenges did you face this month? How can you overcome them?

Challenges	Adjustments

Sleep and Rest

Set specific sleep-related goals for the month (i.e., "achieve 7-8 hours of sleep per night," "improve sleep quality")

New treatments

List the steps you're taking to improve sleep (i.e., "reducing screen time before bed."

Sleep Hygiene Practices

How well are you achieving your sleep goals? What adjustments might be needed?

Tracking Progress

Diet and Nutrition

What are your nutritional goals for this month? (, i.e., "increase vegetable intake."

Dietary Goals

Are you following a specific meal plan or dietary approach?

Meal Planning

Track any changes in energy levels, digestion, or overall well-being related to diet.

Montioring and Adjustments

Recommendations and Resources

List any books or resources recommended by healthcare providers, friends, or family.

Books to Read

Note any courses or workshops you plan to attend this month related to health and wellness.

Courses or Workshops

Record any new insights or recommendations received this month and how you plan to implement them.

New Learning

Reflection and Adjustment

Reflect on your health journey this month. What worked well? What didn't? What surprised you?

Monthly Reflection

Based on this month's experiences, what changes do you need to make to your health plan moving forward?

Adjustments for Next Month

Visit **www.theoprodromitis.com/thewellnessjournal** to access forms for additional Monthly Action Plans and other sections included in this journal, as well as health-related resources and documentation.

www.ingramcontent.com/pod-product-compliance
Lightning Source LLC
Chambersburg PA
CBHW080425030426
42335CB00020B/2590